W0091861

Hypertension in Elderly People

Ken Woodhouse, MRCP FRCP MD
Professor of Geriatric Medicine

and

Juanita Pascual, MB BS MRCP
Consultant Physician in Care of the Elderly

University Department of Geriatric Medicine
University of Wales College of Medicine
Cardiff

MARTIN DUNITZ

Although every effort has been made to ensure that the drug doses and other information are presented accurately in this publication, the ultimate responsibility rests with the prescribing physician. Neither the publishers nor the authors can be held responsible for errors or for any other consequences arising from the use of information contained herein.

© Martin Dunitz Ltd 1996

First published in the United Kingdom in 1996 by

Martin Dunitz Ltd
The Livery House
7–9 Pratt Street
London NW1 0AE

A CIP record for this book is available from the British Library.

ISBN 1-85317-324-X

Printed and bound in Spain by Cayfosa

Contents

Acknowledgements

Figures 1–3, 5, 8, and 13–17 are reproduced with kind permission from Beevers DG, MacGregor GA. *Hypertension in Practice*. 2nd edn. Martin Dunitz, 1995.

Figure 4 is reproduced courtesy of Dr John Wingate, City Hospital, Birmingham.

Figure 6 and 7 are reproduced courtesy of Dr David Perkin, Charing Cross Hospital, London.

Figure 9 is reproduced with kind permission from Swales JD, Sever PS, Peart S. *Clinical Atlas of Hypertension*. Gower Medical Publishing, 1991.

Figure 10–12 are reproduced courtesy of Mr Colin Clements, King's College Hospital, London.

Introduction

The elderly population, particularly the 'very elderly' (over 80 years), is growing rapidly in most developed and many developing countries. Hypertension is a common disorder in all age groups, and is particularly prevalent in the elderly. Depending on the definition used, it has been variously estimated that between 25% and over 50% of the elderly (those over 65) may suffer from this disorder. In the large longitudinal study of ageing undertaken in Gothenberg, Sweden, hypertension treatment was being given to 26% of the over-seventies.

High blood pressure is a crucially important disorder; it is the single most important modifiable risk factor for some of the most common disabling disorders in the elderly, and some of the diseases responsible for the majority of deaths, in particular cerebrovascular and cardiovascular disease.

This book addresses some of the most important issues surrounding blood pressure and its treatment in the elderly, namely:

- Do the benefits of treatment outweigh the risks?

- Should we decide on treatment based on levels of systolic blood pressure, diastolic blood pressure, or both?

- Does better control mean better outcome?

- Does 'overtreatment', that is, lowering the blood pressure too much, result in worse outcomes?

- How should hypertension be diagnosed and managed in the elderly?

- What therapeutic options, pharmacological and non-pharmacological, are available?

Definitions

Various groups have used different definitions of hypertension, and this has complicated studies in this area. For instance, many studies use a systolic/diastolic blood pressure level of >140/90 mmHg as the defining point; the European Working Party on Hypertension in the Elderly used >160/90, the Framingham study >160/95, and so on. Not all studies have tried to compensate for 'white coat' hypertension – that is, blood pressure elevated at the first clinic visit. Even worse, the problems of measurement itself – poor technique in taking blood pressure, different cuff sizes, the known problems of random–zero machines, and the problem of non-compliant brachial arteries – were not appreciated at all in early studies.

The best working definition of hypertension is probably that of the European Working Party on Hypertension in the Elderly:

'An average systolic blood pressure greater than 160 mmHg, or average diastolic blood pressure greater than or equal to 90 mmHg on three consecutive visits constitutes a diagnosis of hypertension.'

Systolic hypertension may be defined as a sustained systolic blood pressure of greater than 160 mmHg, with a diastolic blood pressure of 90 mmHg or less.

The rise in blood pressure that occurs with age is well documented in industrialized countries (Figure 1). In the United States and Europe, systolic blood pressure rises throughout the lifespan of the individual. Diastolic blood pressure rises until about 60 years of age, either levelling off or even gradually decreasing after age 70. Cross-sectional studies show that in young adulthood men tend to have higher blood pressure than

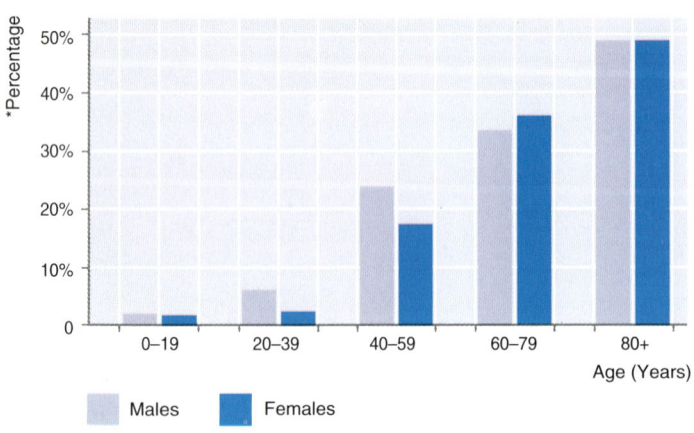

Figure 1
Prevalance of hypertension by age group in industrialized countries. (*percentage of population with SBP ≥ 160 mmHg, DBP ≥ 95 mmHg).

women, but that the age-related rise in blood pressure in females is rather greater than in males so that, by 60 years old, women tend to have a slightly higher blood pressure than men (Figure 2). However, it has been suggested that one reason for this may be premature death among men with raised blood pressure, resulting in a 'selective survival effect' in men who had lower blood pressure at a younger age.

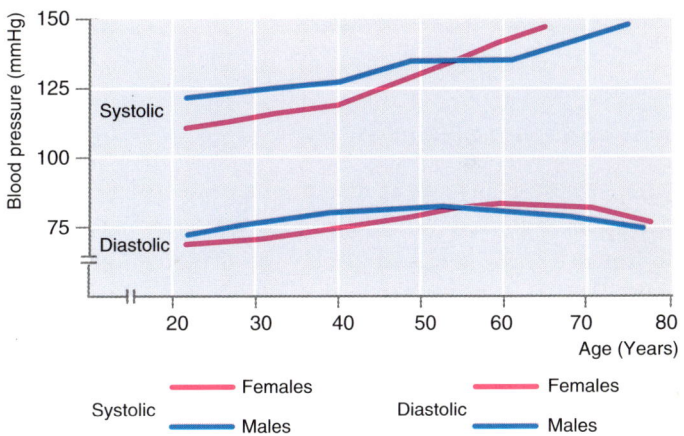

Figure 2
Change in blood pressure with age among men and women.

Some studies have suggested that age *per se* is not necessarily the main underlying cause of the age-related rise in blood pressure. For example, some populations in developing countries do not exhibit the same rise as seen in developed countries (Figure 3); although when genetically similar populations become urbanized, the typical 'Western' age-related rise in blood pressure is seen, suggesting that some factor related to industrialization – such as diet, weight, smoking, alcohol or stress – may contribute more than ageing *per se*.

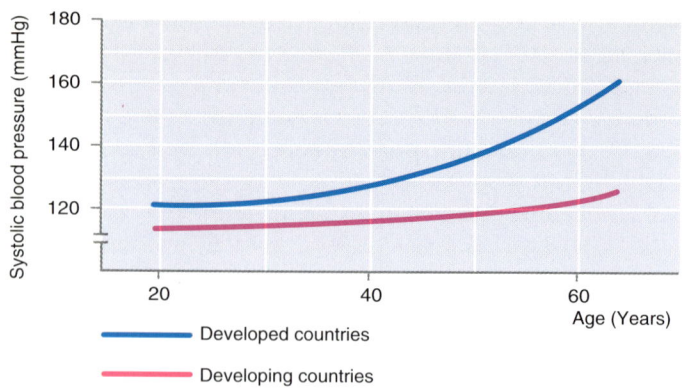

Figure 3
Changes in blood pressure in developed and developing countries.

Other factors which may influence the age-related increase in blood pressure include pre-existing hypertension and race. Those who are hypertensive in younger age are likely to show a more marked increase in blood pressure with ageing if they do not succumb earlier to the complications of the disease.

Population subgroup	Men (%)	Women (%)	Total (%)
African-American	71.6	71.9	71.8
White	54.9	51.2	52.9
Mexican-American	56.9	53.1	54.9

Table 1
Prevalence of hypertension in ethnic populations aged 65–74 years in the United States. Hypertension is defined here as the average of 3 blood pressure measurements ≥ 140 mmHg systolic and ≥ 90 mmHg diastolic on a single occasion or as taking antihypertensive medication. (National High Blood Pressure Education Working Group.)

In the United States in particular, those of African descent have higher blood pressure than whites after age 30, and this is particularly marked in black women. Indeed, past the age of 55, over 70% of black women have hypertension (using the definition of blood pressure >140/90 mmHg) (Table 1).

The true prevalence of hypertension in the elderly is rather difficult to pin down; quoted figures vary greatly depending on the actual level of blood pressure taken to indicate hypertension, and the number of times the blood pressure was measured. Table 2 illustrates this problem.

Age range	Blood pressure cutoff	Number of visits	Prevalence of hypertension (%)
65–74	>140/90	1	64
	>160/95	1	45
60–69	DBP >90	2	14
60+ (whites)	SBP > 160, DBP < 90*	3	
60–79			7
70–79			11
80–89			18

SBP, systolic blood pressure; DBP, diastolic blood pressure.

Table 2
Estimates of the prevalence of hypertension in the elderly.
*Systolic hypertension.

Pathophysiology

A large number of changes have been reported in a variety of body systems in the elderly which may relate to the development of raised levels of blood pressure. These include changes in:

- The vascular structure itself

- Neurovascular and adrenergic responses

- Neurohumoral mechanisms

- The kidney and adrenals

The exact role of these changes in the pathogenesis of hypertension as a disease is unclear, and it is certain that a complex series of interactions of all of these factors is important.

Morphological changes

One of the cardinal changes of ageing in any organ containing connective tissue is a decrease in elasticity. This is particularly obvious in wrinkled skin, but also occurs in the lungs and, not least, in the arterial tree. There is now good evidence that with age, the aorta becomes progressively elongated and more tortuous, its diameter and volume increase and its distensibility and compliance fall markedly. One result of this is a greater resistance to systolic ejection of blood from the heart, accompanied by a rise in systolic blood pressure and an increase in pulse wave velocity and pulse pressure. These changes, more than anything else, are probably responsible for the high prevalence of systolic hypertension in the older person.

Neurovascular function

The autonomic nervous system has been studied extensively in older people. For example, it is known that plasma noradrenaline concentrations increase with age, a finding which interestingly is less apparent in those with hypertension; again, the significance of this is uncertain.

It has been well documented that β_1 adrenergic systems are impaired in the elderly; the best demonstration of this being the decreased cardiac chronotropic response to infused isoprenaline and the decrease in blood vessel dilatation in response to intra-arterial infusions of the same drug. By contrast, studies of α_1 adrenergic mechanisms have led to less conclusive results. In general, it is felt that these systems do not undergo significant changes in the ageing process. These alterations in adrenergic response have led to the theory that reduced β_1-mediated vascular dilatation, coupled with a maintained α_1 adrenergic vasoconstriction are, at least in part, responsible for the increased peripheral vascular resistance seen in elderly hypertensives, and may have a role in the pathogenesis of the condition.

Kidney and adrenals

A variety of changes have been reported in renal function in the elderly and in important humoral activities acting on the kidney. These are summarized in Table 3. Renal blood flow falls with age, and glomerular sclerosis is more prevalent. Sodium homeostasis is poor, reflected by a reduction in the ability to concentrate and excrete sodium. Glomerular filtration rate does fall, on average, as does tubular function, but the rate of fall varies considerably between individuals, little change occurring in some but marked reduction in others.

Plasma atrial natriuretic peptide levels rise with age; this is a feature of ageing, or rather age-associated renal changes, and does not simply reflect the increased prevalence of hypertension in the elderly. However, the significance of these differences is unclear.

Parameter	Change
• Glomerulus	Sclerosis
• Renal blood flow	Decreased
• Glomerular filtration	Decreased
• Tubular function	Decreased
• Plasma atrial natriuretic peptide	Raised
• Plasma renin	Decreased

Table 3
Renal homeostasis and ageing.

Plasma renin levels fall with age, both in the basal stage and in response to sodium restriction. Similarly, the elderly have a decreased renin response at any given level of salt intake. Depsite these changes in plasma renin, and the low occurrence of elevated plasma renin levels in the old, there is no doubt that angiotensin converting enzyme (ACE) inhibitors are extremely effective therapeutic agents in treating raised blood pressure in the elderly (as will be described later); this suggests that the renin–angiotensin mechanism still has an important part to play in maintaining high blood pressure in older people.

Consequences of hypertension

Cardiovascular disease and cerebrovascular disease are major causes of morbidity and mortality in the elderly (Figures 4–7). Over half the deaths occurring in those over 65 years are attributable to one of these causes. An enormous amount of epidemiological data are now available on risk factors for these diseases. The elderly are different from the young in many ways, and important variables such as smoking and family history, while still relevant in elderly people, become less significant whereas hypertension remains a crucial and modifiable risk factor in older people. Traditionally, doctors tended to regard **diastolic blood pressure** as the most important parameter when deciding whether or not to treat hypertension. However, it is now known that **systolic blood pressure** is more important in determining subsequent cardiovascular events. For people aged between 55 and 74 years with isolated systolic hypertension, all-cause morbidity doubles and deaths from cardiovascular disease are elevated twofold in men and fourfold in women.

In addition to death from ischaemic heart disease, the effects of increased blood pressure on ventricular function are equally important. Recent evidence from the Framingham study shows that isolated systolic hypertension and left ventricular hyper-

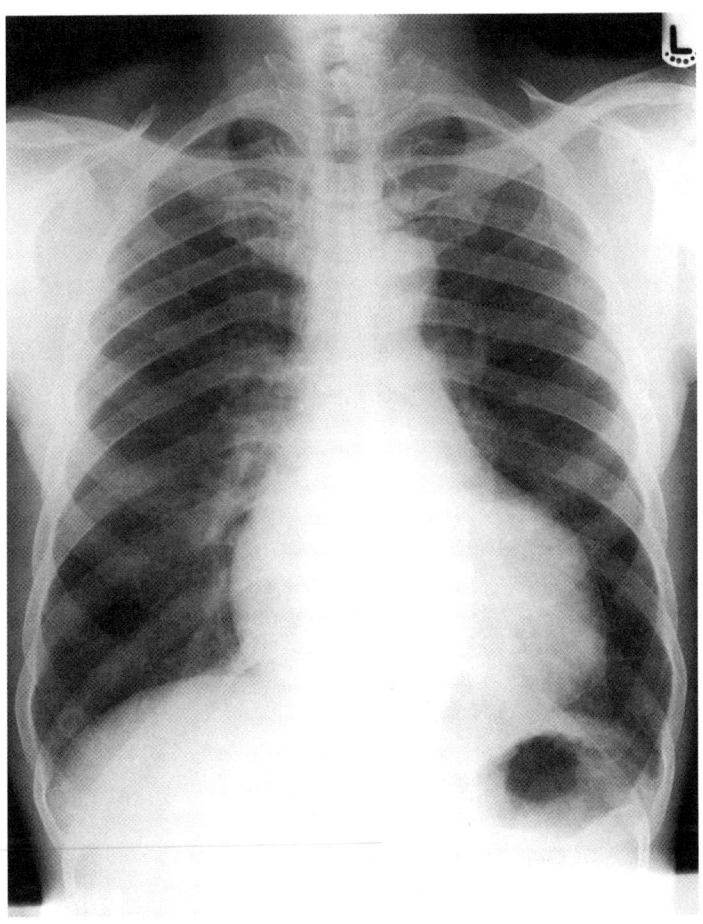

Figure 4
Chest X-ray showing cardiomegaly with upper lobe blood diversion and early interstitial pulmonary oedema.

trophy are strongly associated in the elderly, and up to 60% of elderly hypertensives have left ventricular hypertrophy. This is accompanied by the risk of arrhythmias, diastolic dysfunction

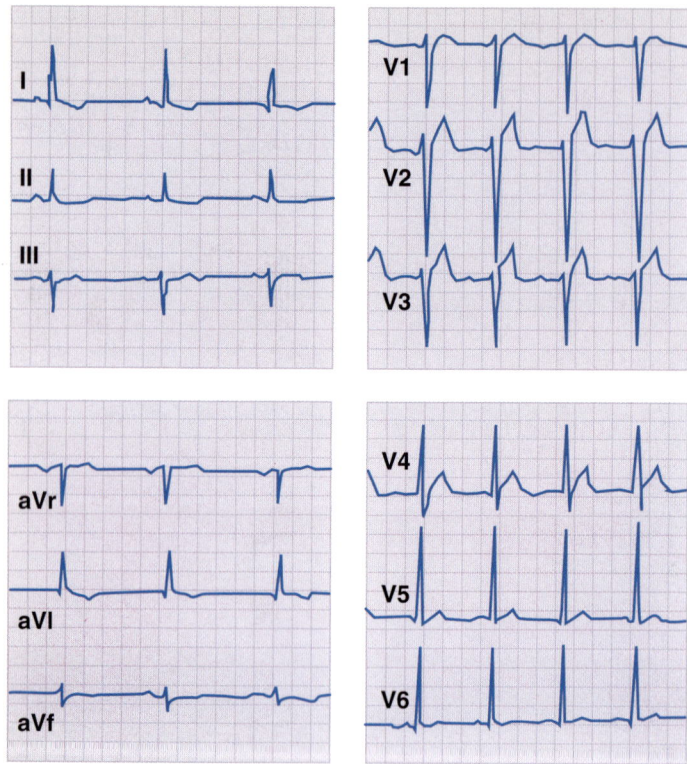

Figure 5
ECG of a patient with left ventricular hypertrophy.

(which may account for up to 30% of heart failure in older women), and frank congestive cardiac failure with all of its associated impact on quality of life.

Stroke and other cerebrovascular events are much more frequent in those with systolic and/or diastolic hypertension. Men with isolated systolic hypertension have a fourfold increased risk of stroke; in women, the risk is increased twofold. This

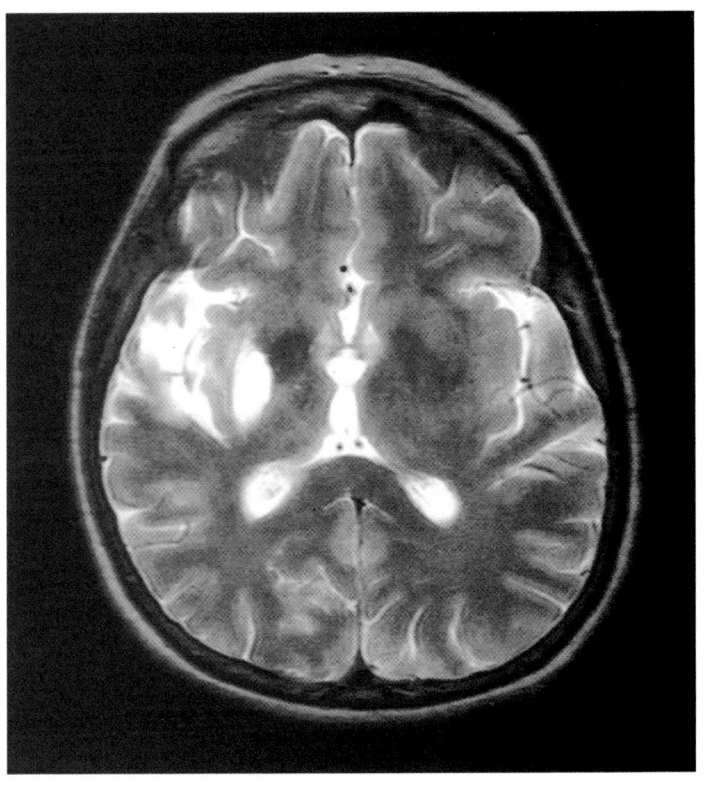

Figure 6
MRI showing mature infarct in the left middle cerebral artery territory.

increased risk does not lessen with age, and is also more apparent at increasing levels of blood pressure. Equally important in terms of morbidity and social impact is the occurrence of multi-infarct dementia; it is clear that this condition is substantially more common in elderly hypertensives.

More controversial is the role of elevated blood pressure in determining morbidity and mortality in the very elderly. Up to

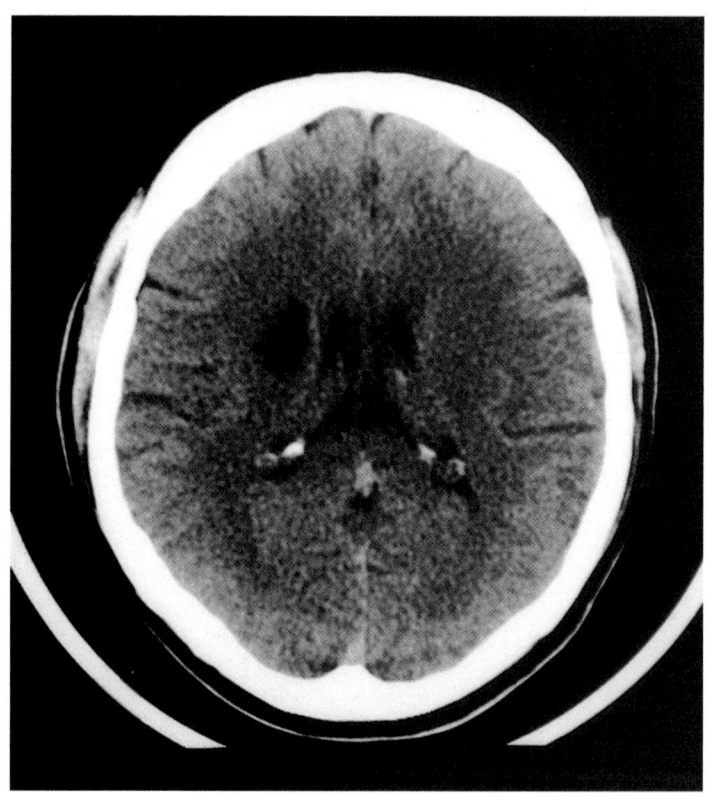

Figure 7
CT scan showing infarct in the left corpus striatum.

the age of 75–80 years the associations described above are incontrovertible, but there is some evidence that among the very old, high levels of blood pressure may not confer such an adverse outcome. For example, in one study in Finland, Mattila and colleagues showed that all-cause mortality was actually lower in those with a systolic blood pressure >160 mmHg and diastolic blood pressure >90 mmHg. Many authors have discussed these findings at length and it may well be that those with a lower blood pressure in this study reflected a sub-group with established cardiovascular disease, who subsequently had a higher mortality. These findings do complicate the approach to treatment of elevated levels of blood pressure in very elderly people, presenting dilemmas which can only be answered by carefully controlled clinical trials.

Diagnosis and investigation

Blood pressure variability is a well-recognized phenomenon and is influenced by a number of factors (Table 4). Indeed, over one-third of the elderly population may be classified as hypertensive if only one blood pressure measurement is performed. Because of this, and the fact that antihypertensive treatment is not without its problems, accurate assessment of blood pressure is required before any treatment is initiated.

- Blood pressure varies minute-to-minute due to changes in respiration and vasomotor tone
- Mental and physical activity increase blood pressure
- Blood pressure falls post-prandially and during sleep
- Hypertensive patients have a greater blood pressure variability
- Blood pressure is higher when taken:

    —at a clinic

    —by a doctor rather than another healthcare professional ('white coat' effect)
- Blood pressure tends to fall with time after repeated measurements – especially in the elderly (e.g. intervention trials of hypertension show a decrease of around 5 mmHg in the placebo group at three months)

Table 4
Factors influencing blood pressure variability.

Measurement of blood pressure

As well as the factors listed above, which can lead to variation in measured blood pressure levels, the measurer can also be responsible for erroneous or variable blood pressure measurement. The following are recommended:

- Blood pressure should be measured on at least three separate occasions over 2–3 months

- Measurements should be taken after 10 minutes rest, sitting or supine

- Blood pressure should be measured in both arms (10% of elderly people have a difference between arms of >10 mmHg)

- Use a large enough cuff to avoid falsely elevated blood pressure readings

The role of 24 hour ambulatory blood pressure monitoring

Most studies on the benefit of treating elderly hypertensives are based on standard blood pressure measurements rather than 24 hour ambulatory levels, and there are currently no criteria for 24 hour ambulatory measurement as regards diagnosing and treating the elderly. In addition, 24 hour ambulatory blood pressure monitoring requires expensive equipment which is not widely available for routine use.

A particular use of 24 hour ambulatory blood pressure monitoring is in distinguishing those patients who display the 'white coat' phenomenon from those who have sustained hypertension at home as well as in the clinic. As a research tool, 24 hour blood pressure monitoring may in future identify those elderly patients with a higher cardiovascular risk. A recent study suggests that hypertensive elderly patients whose blood pressure does not fall significantly at night have a higher incidence of cardiovascular disease.

Investigations

Baseline investigations of hypertensives include:

- Full blood count
- Urea, electrolytes and creatinine
- Urate
- Glucose
- Chest X-ray
- Electrocardiogram (ECG)

Investigations of hypertensives of all ages are aimed at:

- Assessing end-organ damage
- Identifying associated conditions and risk factors which contribute to cardiovascular and other hypertension-associated morbidity
- Determining whether there are any reversible secondary causes of hypertension

Assessing end-organ damage

The consequences of hypertension (Figures 8–12) are most marked in the heart, kidneys, eyes and brain. In the elderly, however, it may be difficult to distinguish the effects of hypertension on these organs from those of 'normal ageing' and other systemic illness.

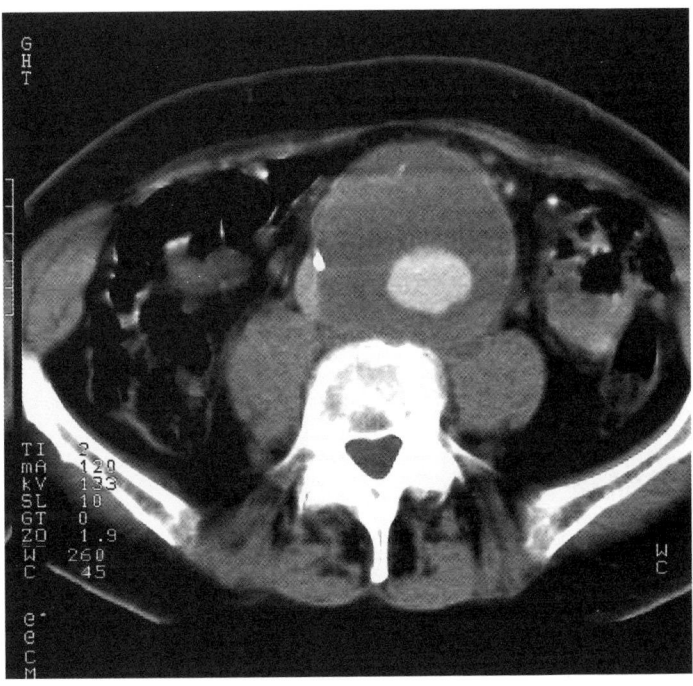

Figure 8
CT scan showing abdominal aortic aneurysm.

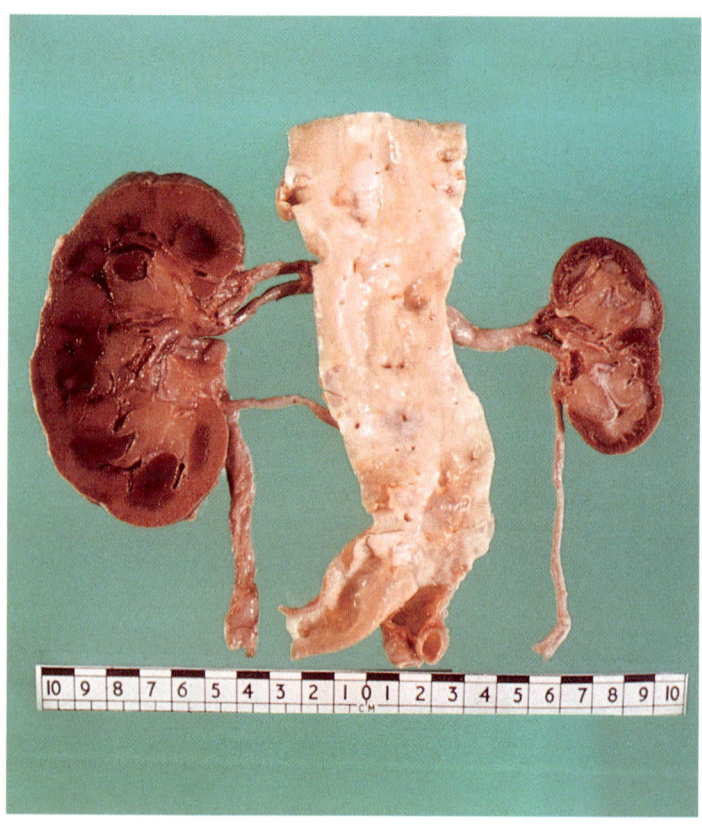

Figure 9
Atheroma and left renal artery stenosis.

Fundoscopy is useful to identify the severe retinopathy associated with malignant hypertension and may also disclose concomitant diabetic retinopathy – it should therefore be performed
on all patients at initial assessment. The fundoscopic changes
associated with mild hypertension are indistinguishable from
those of ageing and are not therefore helpful in management.

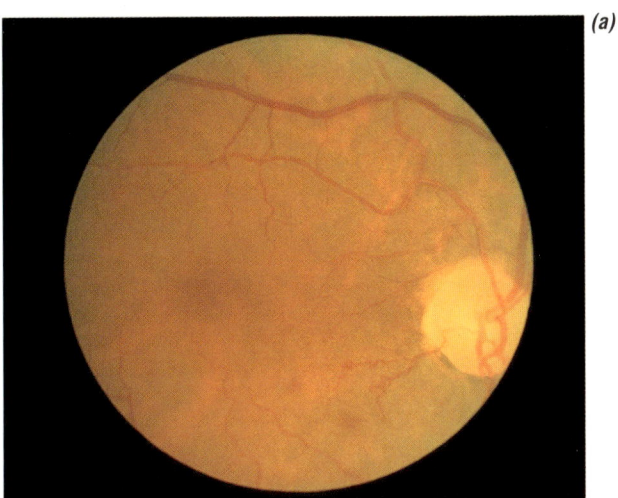

(a)

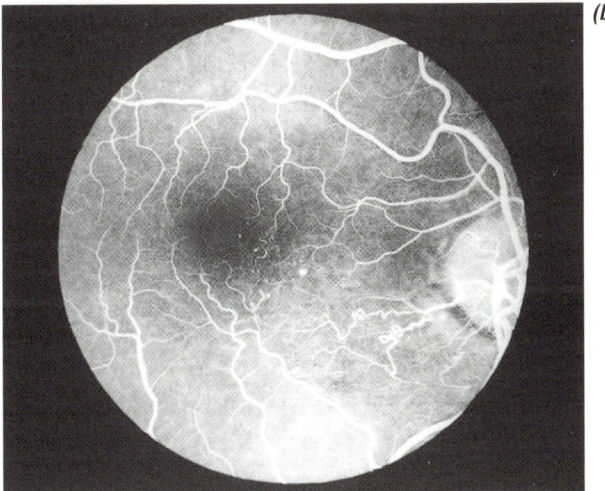

(b)

Figure 10
(a) Right eye showing tortuous vessels supero-temporal to the optic disc and some microaneurysms close to the fovea, possibly a microvascular occlusion secondary to hypertension. (b) Fluorescein angiogram in the arteriovenous phase of the same patient, showing the tortuous vessels, microaneurysms and dilated capillaries on the nasal side of the foveal arcade. There is also some capillary 'drop out' indicating early ischaemia.

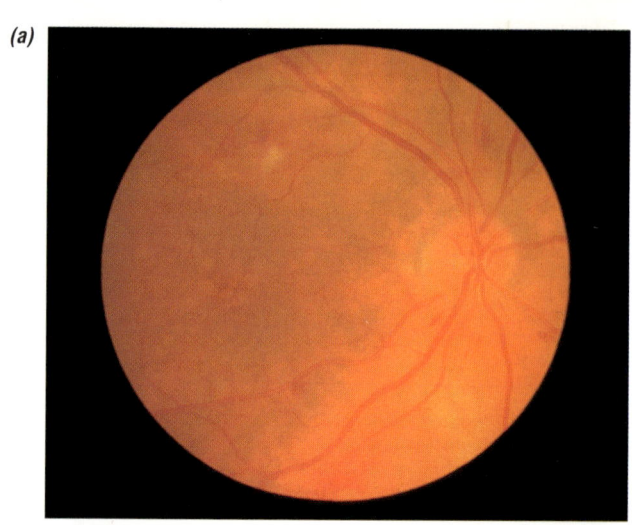

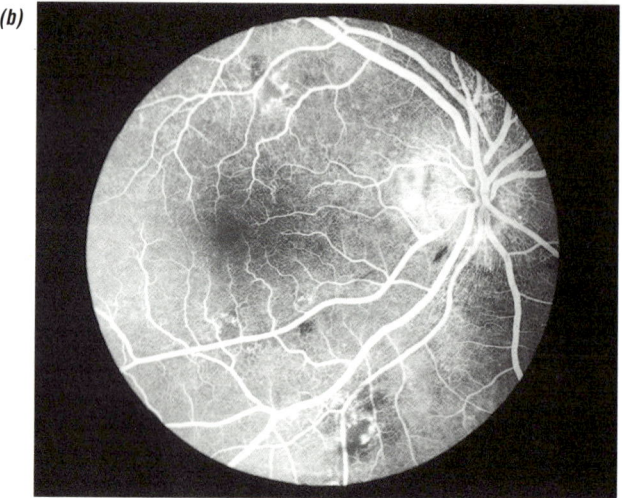

Figure 11
(a) Right eye showing some scattered haemorrhages and a cotton wool spot; there are some age-related drusen at the macula. *(b)* Fluorescein angiogram in the arteriovenous phase of the same patient, showing the cotton wool spot clearly visible in the supero-temporal quadrant.

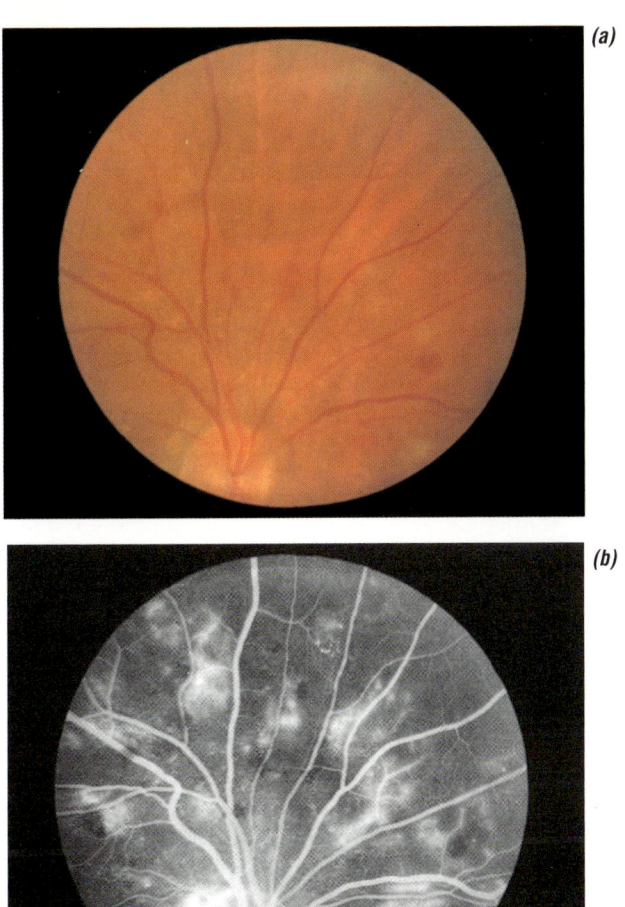

Figure 12
(a) Left eye of the same patient as in Figure 11, showing numerous cotton wool spots and haemorrhages supero-nasal to the disc. *(b)* Fluorescein angiogram in the arteriovenous phase showing masking from the haemorrhages and cotton wool spots. There is leakage from and staining of vessels as they cross poorly perfused areas of the retina. A few microaneurysms can be seen at the top of the picture.

Hypertension is a risk factor for the development of left ventricular hypertrophy, congestive cardiac failure and coronary heart disease. Left ventricular hypertrophy and impairment may help to identify a high risk group who should be targeted for more aggressive therapy. However, the most sensitive means of identifying these patients is by echocardiography. Unfortunately, this technique is not always available and, moreover, elderly patients, because of anatomical changes, often make poor echo subjects. At present echocardiography cannot be recommended as a baseline assessment for all elderly hypertensives.

The increased incidence of peripheral vascular disease and aortic aneurysm also needs to be borne in mind when assessing elderly hypertensives. Peripheral pulses should be examined, the abdomen palpated, and bruits auscultated for, in all patients.

As far as the kidney is concerned it can be difficult in the elderly to determine whether hypertension has occurred secondarily to renal disease or is a primary initiating or exacerbating factor (Table 5). In essential hypertension the kidney shows changes consistent with an acceleration of normal physiological ageing. Atheromatous renal artery stenosis is the only major cause of secondary hypertension in the elderly and, as such, is the main secondary cause which should be actively sought and excluded (Table 6).

Cardiovascular risk factors and conditions associated with hypertension

A higher than average incidence of diabetes, hyperlipidaemia and gout is well recognized among hypertensives. However, while serum glucose and urate are useful baseline investigations, the value of serum cholesterol levels in predicting cardiovascular mortality and influencing it by treatment has not been established in the elderly. At present the role of lipid estimations in the treatment of hyperlipidaemic elderly hypertensives remains a debatable issue.

- Abrupt onset
- Rapid progression
- Smoking
- Blood pressure difficult to control
- Evidence of other atherosclerotic disease, e.g. peripheral vascular and coronary artery disease

Table 5
Factors suggesting renal artery stenosis as a secondary cause of hypertension.

- Abdominal ultrasound (inequality of renal size)
- Intravenous urography

More specific tests include:

Captopril isotope renography

Intravenous digital subtraction angiography

Differential renal renin determinations

If these tests are suggestive, arteriography with a view to angioplasty should be considered

Table 6
Screening for renal artery stenosis.

Assessment of lifestyle risk factors including obesity, exercise, alcohol, smoking and sodium and potassium intake should be undertaken and appropriate non-pharmacological advice given to each individual. There is good evidence that modification of lifestyle factors can lead to a significant reduction in blood pressure without recourse to drug therapy (see pages 40–43).

Treating hypertension in the elderly – is it worthwhile?

It is clearly established that hypertension is a significant risk factor for cardiovascular morbidity and mortality in the elderly – however, this does not necessarily imply that the treatment of hypertension is going to be beneficial.

Until recently the only data available on the benefits of treating elderly hypertensives were derived from sub-group analysis of larger population studies. The information derived from these studies was limited as they were not aimed specifically at the elderly and therefore the number of patients in the over 65 age group was small. In the past few years, however, a number of studies have been published looking specifically at the effects of antihypertensive treatment in the elderly and the results to date are, on the whole, encouraging (Figure 13).

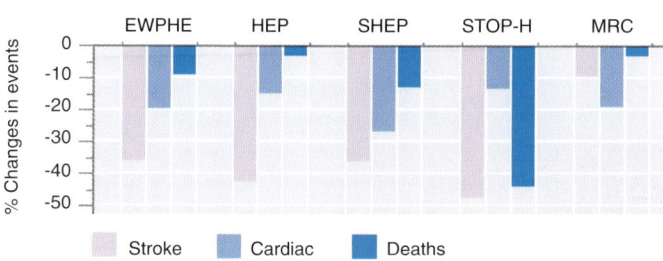

Figure 13
Comparison of six clinical trials showing the decreases shown in stroke, cardiac events and death.

Randomized intervention trials in the elderly

European Working Party on Hypertension in the Elderly (EWHPE) Trial	
Number of subjects	840
Age group	60+ (mean age 72)
Treatment tested	*hydrochlorthiazide and triamterene versus placebo*
Study design	recruited from outpatient clinics double blind, randomized followed up for $4\frac{1}{2}$ years
Blood pressure criteria	>160/90 mmHg
Results	• significant reduction in cardiovascular mortality and deaths from myocardial infarction • non-significant reduction in cerebrovascular deaths and overall mortality • main benefits seen in those aged less than 80 years and with moderate reduction in blood pressure
Reference	Amery A et al. Lancet 1985 volume i pp 1349–54

Hypotensive Elderly Patients (HEP) Trial

Number of subjects	884
Age group	60–79
Treatment tested	*atenolol ± bendrofluazide versus placebo*
Study design	recruited from general practices followed up for $4\frac{1}{2}$ years
Blood pressure criteria	>170/105 mmHg
Results	• significant reduction in fatal and total strokes • non-significant reduction in cardiovascular mortality • no effect on incidence of myocardial infarction
Reference	Coope J, Warrender TS. British Medical Journal 1986 volume 293 pp 1145–51

Systolic Hypertension in the Elderly Project (SHEP)

Number of subjects	4736
Age group	>60 (mean age 72)
Treatment tested	*chorthalidone versus placebo (chlorthalidone switched to atenolol or reserpine if ineffective)*
Study design	double blind, randomized followed for 5 years
Blood pressure criteria	systolic >160 mmHg diastolic <90 mmHg

Results
(Figure 14)
	• significant reductions in:
	  —stroke incidence
	  —myocardial infarction incidence
	  —cardiovascular deaths
	  —cardiovascular events
	  —overall mortality
	• equal benefit seen in those aged over 80 as well as under 80 years

Reference	SHEP Cooperative Research Group. Journal of the American Medical Association 1991 volume 265 pp 3255–64

Swedish Trial in Old Patients with Hypertension (STOP–H)	
Number of subjects	1627
Age group	70–84
Treatment tested	*thiazide versus β-blockers versus placebo*
Study design	double blind, randomized followed for 25 months
Blood pressure criteria	systolic >180 mmHg diastolic 90–110 mmHg
Results (Table 7)	• significant reduction in: —fatal and non-fatal strokes —cardiovascular events —cardiovascular and total mortality • non-significant reduction in incidence of myocardial infarction
Reference	Dahlof B et al. Lancet 1991 volume 338 pp 1281–5

Medical Research Council trial of treatment of hypertension in older adults

Number of subjects	4396
Age group	65–75
Treatment tested	*atenolol versus hydrochlorthiazide plus amiloride versus placebo*
Study design	single blind, randomized
Blood pressure criteria	systolic >180 mmHg diastolic 90–110 mmHg

Results (Figure 15)	• significant reduction in:
	  —stroke
	  —cardiovascular events
	  —coronary events
	  only in the diuretic group
	• no significant reduction in end-points seen with atenolol

Reference	MRC Working Party. British Medical Journal 1992 vol 304 pp 405–12

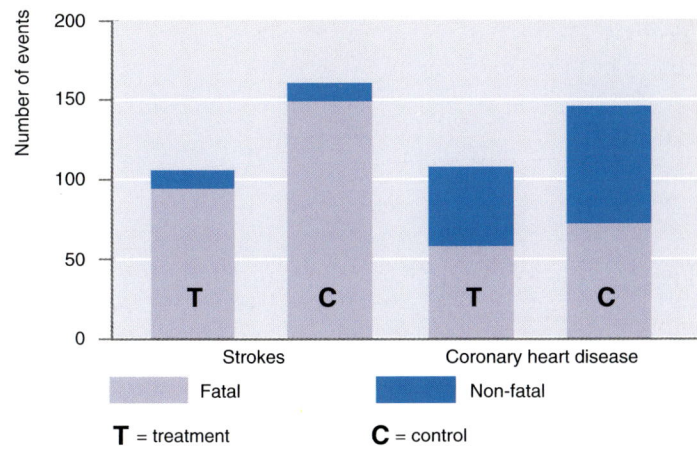

Figure 14
Results of treatment in the SHEP study.

	Treatment	Placebo
Myocardial infarction		
All	14.4	16.5
Fatal	3.4	4.5
Stroke		
All	16.8	31.3
Fatal	2.3	8.3
Other cardiovascular deaths	1.7	3.4
Total deaths	20.2	35.4

Table 7
Findings in the STOP–H trial (events per 1000 patients per year).

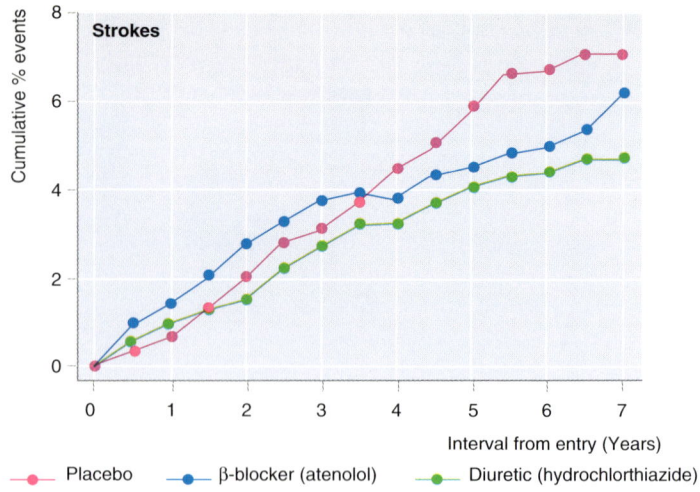

Figure 15
Effects of treatment in the MRC trial on frequency of strokes and coronary heart disease.

	Criteria	Treatment
Uncomplicated mild hypertension	SBP 160–185 mmHg or DBP 95–110 mmHg	Non-pharmacological treatment with 3–6 months follow-up
Sustained hypertension after 3–6 months as above	SBP >160 mmHg or DBP >90 mmHg	Initiate drug therapy
Moderate/severe hypertension	SBP >185 mmHg, DBP >110 mmHg, or complications, e.g. heart failure	Initiate drug therapy immediately

Table 8
Suggested guidelines for antihypertensive treatment in the elderly.

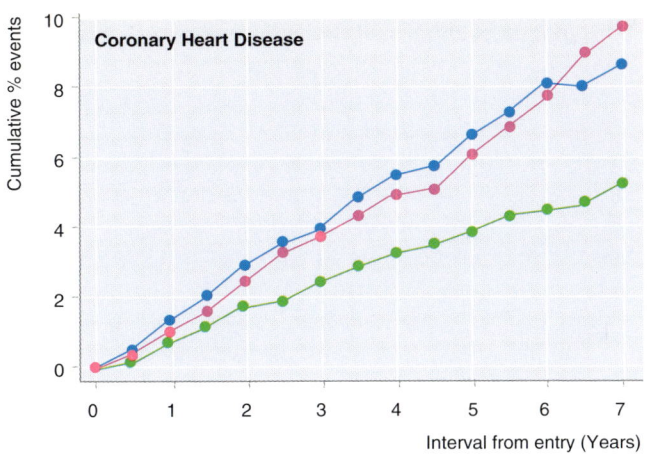

Coronary Heart Disease

Cumulative % events

Interval from entry (Years)

What level of blood pressure should we treat?

The elderly are a diverse group with individuals varying greatly in terms of physical frailty and co-existing medical illnesses – it is therefore difficult to apply rigid criteria for commencing anti-hypertensive treatment in a given individual. Suggested general guidelines are shown in Table 8.

What age to treat and for how long?

The EWPHE trial showed no benefit in those aged over 80; however, the SHEP and STOP–H trials did. Unfortunately, there are few data on the benefits of treating the very elderly, i.e. those aged over 80. In general, we can say at present that treating patients up to the age of 80 years is beneficial, and that treatment in those who are able to tolerate it up to age 85 is reasonable.

As far as those elderly hypertensives who have already been on antihypertensive treatment for some years are concerned, a number of factors must be taken into account (Table 9). In those patients with sustained hypertension and evidence of end-organ damage, such as cardiac failure and cerebrovascular disease, continued treatment is desirable, but drug therapy is not without its problems, particularly in the frail elderly. It is always important to maintain regular monitoring and follow-up in order to avoid end-organ damage occurring unnoticed. It may be possible to withdraw antihypertensive treatment, particularly in those who are well controlled on single drug regimes, and studies suggest that 5–50% of patients can have their treatment successfully discontinued while remaining normotensive.

- More than one drug required to control blood pressure

- High pre-treatment blood pressure levels

- Obesity

- Short duration of treatment (e.g. 1–2 years)

- Evidence of left ventricular hypertrophy

- Lack of regular follow-up and dietary and other lifestyle advice

---

Table 9
Factors adversely influencing successful withdrawal of antihypertensive therapy.

How far should blood pressure be reduced?

There is some evidence that lowering blood pressure too far can have adverse effects on morbidity and mortality, particularly in those individuals with pre-existing ischaemic heart disease. Both the Framingham study and the EHWPE study revealed a U-shaped relationship between diastolic blood pressure and mortality. The lowest mortality is seen in the diastolic blood pressure range 79–94 mmHg, and it would therefore be prudent in monitoring treatment not to lower blood pressure below 70 mmHg. The data on target systolic blood pressure levels are less clear, although current evidence suggests that lowering systolic blood pressure below 140 mmHg is unlikely to be beneficial.

Treating isolated systolic hypertension

The results of the SHEP trial have clearly shown benefit in treating isolated systolic hypertension in the elderly up to at least the mid-eighties. It is not clear, however, how long treatment should be continued or if it is of value in even older subjects.

Treating hypertension after stroke

Although antihypertensive treatment reduces the incidence of a first stroke, current studies suggest that it appears not to greatly influence the risk of second or recurrent stroke. It is worth remembering that in the first few days after stroke blood pressure often rises to high levels, but that abrupt lowering of blood pressure in such circumstances can lead to infarct extension, due to stroke associated changes in regional blood flow and cerebral autoregulation. Treatment in this situation is rarely indicated, unless blood pressure is 'malignant', with hypertensive encephalopathy present. Blood pressure should be simply observed and allowed to fall naturally over a number of days, with antihypertensive therapy initiated at 1–2 weeks if deemed necessary.

Non-pharmacological approaches to treatment

Few studies have examined the effect of non-pharmacological approaches on blood pressure in the elderly. However, studies performed mostly on younger subjects have shown benefit in terms of modest reductions in blood pressure and mortality from such interventions. It seems reasonable to extrapolate that the elderly will respond equally well to such measures and, in mild hypertension, to try these before instituting drug therapy.

Salt restriction

Lowering dietary salt intake is one of the most widely accepted non-pharmacological approaches to lowering blood pressure. An overview of trials in all age groups found a blood pressure reduction of 3–5 mmHg with varying degrees of salt restriction. A moderate reduction in sodium intake of about 50 mmol/day can be achieved by avoiding salty foods and not adding extra salt to food in cooking or at the table.

A couple of points are worth bearing in mind:

1   The elderly have diminished taste sensation, usually use more salt to counteract the lack of taste, and are therefore poor compliers with low salt diets.

2   Severe salt restriction and continued water intake can lead to severe hyponatraemia.

On the plus side, low salt diets may help to prevent diuretic-induced hypokalaemia and may be of particular value in those patients with congestive cardiac failure.

Potassium intake

A recent trial of elderly hypertensives found that potassium supplementation of 60 mmol/day lowered blood pressure by 6–10 mmHg. This finding is supported by an overview of trials in younger subjects. Dietary advice on increasing consumption of fresh fruit and vegetables can significantly improve potassium intake as well as contributing to a healthier diet.

Weight reduction

The association between obesity and hypertension is well known (Figure 16), and weight reduction has been shown to reduce blood pressure. However, it is worth remembering that compliance with any dietary measures is notoriously poor in the elderly. Lifestyles are mostly well established and the elderly are often reluctant to consider changes.

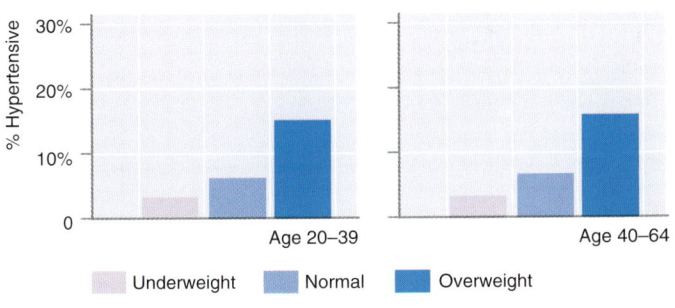

Figure 16
Prevalence of hypertension in relation to weight.

Exercise

Low grade exercise programmes have been shown to be effective in achieving modest blood pressure reductions in elderly patients. Some elderly patients may be precluded from exercise because of concomitant disorders, such as angina or arthritis, but daily exercise has been shown to be feasible in subjects aged over 70 and the benefits often outweigh the difficulties. Low intensity aerobic exercise, such as swimming, cycling or brisk walking should be recommended.

Alcohol

Alcohol is well recognized to have a pressor effect (Figure 17). The relationship between alcohol and blood pressure is not, however, linear – it takes a J-shaped form, with the lowest incidence of hypertension seen in occasional or light drinkers rather than non-drinkers. Reducing alcohol consumption, particularly in heavy drinkers, can lead to substantial falls in blood pressure. As mild alcohol intake appears to have a cardioprotective effect, up to 2 units per day would seem a reasonable recommendation. The maximum recommended weekly intake is shown in Table 10.

	Men	Women
Units/week*	21	14
Beer (pints)	10.5	7
Wine (glass)	21	14
Spirits (measures)	21	14
Sherry, port etc (glass)	21	14
* 1 unit of alcohol is approximately equivalent to 10 g.		

Table 10
Maximum recommended alcohol intake.

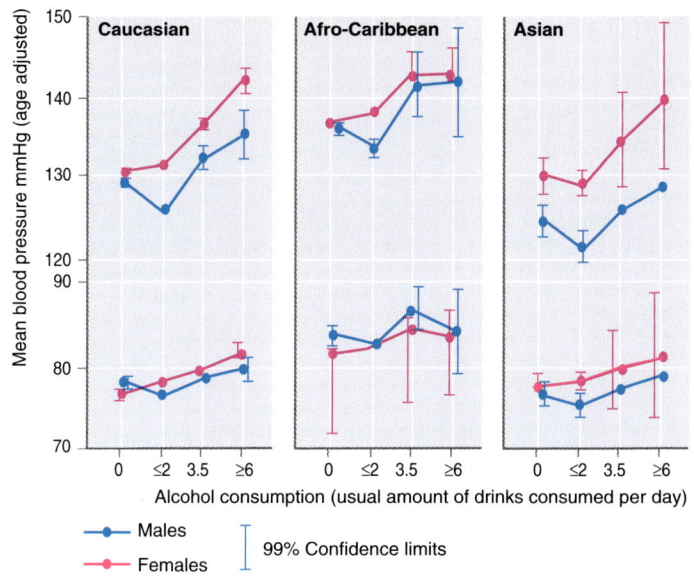

Figure 17
Effects of alcohol intake on blood pressure in three ethnic populations. Data from Kaiser-Permanente Health Insurance Program.

Drug treatment and the elderly

In initiating any drug treatment in an elderly individual, it is essential to bear in mind that the elderly respond differently to drugs compared with their younger counterparts. Moreover, the elderly are a very heterogeneous group in whom chronological age is not a particularly useful guide, and who vary tremendously in their physiological responses, drug handling (elimination and sensitivity), concomitant physical illnesses and general physical frailty. In addition, they are often taking many other prescribed and 'over the counter' drugs. Clearly, all these factors make the action of a given drug on a particular individual much more unpredictable.

In prescribing for the elderly the following factors must be taken into account:

1 Renal function declines with age as does ability to conserve sodium and water:

    —increased potential for toxicity with renally excreted drugs

    —increased susceptibility to diuretic induced hyponatraemia or dehydration

    NB: serum creatinine is not a reliable guide to renal function in the elderly due to the decrease in lean body mass.

2 Liver size and blood flow diminish with age, as does oxidative metabolism.

3 First pass metabolism is decreased, therefore with drugs extensively cleared by this mechanism (e.g. nitrates), an increased amount of the drug reaches the circulation.

4 Physiological changes in target-organ responsiveness occur with ageing, e.g. the number and affinity of β-receptors is reduced causing decreased sensitivity to β-blockers and β-agonists.

5 Changes occur in the homeostatic response, e.g. a decrease in baroreceptor reflexes leads to an increased tendency to postural hypotension.

6 Concomitant illnesses may be exacerbated by antihypertensive treatment:

—thiazides worsen diabetes

—β-blockers worsen asthma, heart failure, and peripheral vascular disease.

7 The elderly are frequently taking other drugs:

—increased potential for drug interactions

—drugs themselves may exacerbate hypertension, e.g. steroids and non-steroidal anti-inflammatory drugs.

It is clear that the elderly have a much greater potential for adverse drug reactions and drug interactions. It is important to tailor drug therapy to each individual patient, taking all these factors and the known adverse effects of giving antihypertensive agents into account. When using a particular drug it is important to titrate the dose, commencing with low doses and avoiding high ones wherever possible, while remaining vigilant for the possible adverse effects.

Thiazide diuretics

Thiazide diuretics have been used in the treatment of hypertension for many years and most intervention studies showing a beneficial effect from treating hypertension in the elderly have used thiazides. Their method of action is incompletely understood, but is partly due to a lowering of intravascular volume and a decrease in peripheral resistance. The SHEP study showed that they are equally effective in treating isolated systolic hypertension, without causing significant postural hypotension.

The adverse effects of thiazide diuretics are well recognized (Table 11). They may initiate or aggravate diabetes, gout, urinary incontinence, prostatic symptoms or impotence. Although thiazides are known to have an adverse effect on plasma lipids, the consequence of this in terms of increased cardiovascular morbidity and mortality remains unproven. There may, however, be a favourable effect from long-term use of thiazides because they elevate serum calcium and may therefore reduce the risk of hip fractures.

- Hypokalaemia
- Hyponatraemia
- Hypomagnesaemia
- Decreased glucose tolerance
- Increased serum urate
- Increased serum creatinine
- Increased low density lipoprotein cholesterol

Table 11
Adverse effects of thiazide diuretics.

When treating hypertension with thiazides it is important to remember that low doses have a similar hypotensive effect to higher doses, with fewer side-effects. If the patient is not responding to low doses there is little or no value in increasing the dose, and another class of drug should be added or substituted. Serum electrolytes should be checked one month after commencing treatment to determine the need for potassium-sparing diuretics. Thiazide diuretics are cheap and have been shown to be effective and well tolerated in large studies of hypertension in the elderly, and their once daily dosage aids compliance. Therefore, they remain one of the first-line agents in treating elderly hypertensives.

β-adrenoceptor blockers

Although the antihypertensive actions of β-blockers are not clearly defined, their effect appears to be mediated by a decrease in cardiac output, while either increasing or having no effect on peripheral resistance. Since the elderly tend to have a lower cardiac output with increased peripheral resistance, and there is also an age-related decrease in β-receptor responsiveness, β-blockers would appear to be unsuitable for treating elderly hypertensives. However, several studies have shown β-blockers to be effective and well tolerated hypotensive agents in the elderly. The adverse effects of β-blockers are well known and Table 12 lists those conditions in which β-blockers should be avoided. However, they may be of value in patients with angina, recent myocardial infarction or supraventricular arrhythmias, provided that left ventricular function is well preserved.

Tiredness, depression, sleep disturbance and effects on concentration and memory have been reported in elderly hypertensives taking β-blockers, particularly the lipophilic β-blockers such as propranolol and metoprolol, which cross the blood-brain barrier. Non-lipophilic β-blockers such as atenolol should therefore be used in preference.

> - Cardiac failure
> - Chronic obstructive airways disease
> - Peripheral vascular disease
> - Asthma
> - Heart block

Table 12
Contraindications to β-blockade.

β-blockers with intrinsic sympathomimetic activity such as pindolol are theoretically advantageous as they maintain cardiac output and preserve left ventricular function – whether they offer any true advantage in clinical practice remains unproven.

Third generation β-blockers such as celiprolol act as weak vasodilators, decreasing peripheral resistance with little effect on cardiac output or heart rate; while theoretically they have advantages over conventional β-blockers in treating the elderly, in practice this has yet to be demonstrated.

Finally, it is worth noting that the Medical Research Council study of antihypertensive treatment in the elderly showed that atenolol, unlike thiazide diuretics, did not reduce fatal strokes or overall cardiovascular events, casting into doubt the use of β-blockers as first-line agents in treating elderly hypertensives.

Calcium antagonists

Calcium channel blockers are well tolerated and effective hypotensive agents in the elderly. They lower blood pressure by reducing peripheral vascular resistance, but although they all act through a similar antihypertensive mechanism they vary in their pharmacological effects. For practical prescribing purposes they can be broadly divided into three groups depending on their relative effects on the heart and blood vessels (Table 13).

There are no clear differences in efficacy among the calcium antagonists. When given alone they control blood pressure in up to 60–80% of patients with mild to moderate hypertension, a rate comparable with other antihypertensive agents. They do not adversely affect renal function and can be used safely in patients with peripheral vascular disease and airways obstruction.

Selection of an appropriate calcium antagonist depends on their particular unwanted effects, especially in relation to the presence

	Negative inotropism	Decreased AV nodal conduction	Peripheral vasodilatation
Verapamil	++	++	++
Diltiazem	+	+	+
Dihydropyridines*	±	no effect	+++/++
(nifedipine, amlodipine, nicardipine, felodipine, isradipine, lacidipine)			

* The dihydropyridines vary from each other in their haemodynamic effects, e.g. amlodipine is not negatively inotropic.

+++ marked effect; ++ moderate effect; + mild effect; ± variable effect.

Table 13
Variation in haemodynamic effects of calcium antagonists on heart and blood vessels.

of concomitant conditions. For example the negative inotropic properties of verapamil, and to a lesser extent diltiazem, can lead to worsening of cardiac failure in patients with impaired left ventricular function. The 'second generation' dihydropyridines (nicardipine, amlodipine, felodipine, isradipine and lacidipine) are claimed to be safer than nifedipine in patients with left ventricular impairment. Most calcium antagonists carry a warning about use with patients with poor cardiac reserve (congestive heart failure); however, there are differences between each of the calcium antagonists. For example, there are now data available clearly demonstrating that amlodipine can be used to treat hypertension or angina without worsening coexsistent mild or moderate congestive heart failure.

Verapamil and diltiazem can cause marked bradycardia in patients with conducting system disease or bradyarrhythmias, and they are therefore contraindicated in patients with heart block or sick sinus syndrome.

Severe hypotension and bradycardia are a significant risk when verapamil is given together with a β-blocker, and this combination should be avoided. Diltiazem may, to a lesser extent, cause similar problems, particularly at higher doses.

All calcium antagonists can cause headache and flushing due to their vasodilator effects. These are most troublesome with the dihydropyridines and are most intense at the times of peak plasma drug concentrations. Reflex tachycardia may occur and can lead to a worsening of anginal symptoms. Amlodipine, with its long half-life, and the modified release preparations may help to reduce these effects by avoiding excessive peaks in plasma concentrations.

Ankle oedema can occur with all the calcium antagonists; it is more common with the dihydropyridines and still seen, if to a lesser extent, with modified release agents or long-acting preparations such as amlodipine.

Calcium antagonists relax smooth muscle and some may worsen oesophageal reflux. Verapamil (and to a lesser extent diltiazem) can cause troublesome constipation.

Urinary frequency and nocturia have been reported with the dihydropyridines, as has gum hypertrophy.

Angiotensin converting enzyme (ACE) inhibitors

ACE inhibitors are effective antihypertensive agents in the elderly. Their benefits in improving morbidity and mortality in patients with both chronic heart failure and heart failure following acute myocardial infarction are now well recognized, and they are therefore clearly drugs of choice in treating elderly hypertensives with concomitant heart failure or evidence of left ventricular impairment. They act by decreasing peripheral resistance and dilating capacitance vessels, while maintaining systemic and regional blood flow.

Caution needs to be exercised when initiating therapy with ACE inhibitors. Marked first-dose hypotension may occur, particularly in those who are hypovolaemic, hyponatraemic or taking diuretics. Diuretic therapy should be withheld at least 24 hours prior to initiating treatment, and a low starting dose should be used, e.g. captopril 6.25 mg daily or enalapril 2.5 mg daily. There is now a large number of ACE inhibitors available for use, and some are being promoted as having a lower incidence of first-dose hypotension. In practice first-dose hypotension can occur with all ACE inhibitors, but this effect may reverse sooner if a short-acting ACE inhibitor such as captopril is used as a test dose. Side-effects associated with ACE inhibitors are listed in Table 14.

ACE inhibitors can elevate potassium levels and all potassium-sparing diuretics should be discontinued prior to initiating treatment to avoid life-threatening hyperkalaemia.

- **First dose hypotension**

  risk ↑ if: age >70
  concomitant heart failure
  dehydration
  taking a diuretic

- **Renal impairment**

  risk ↑ if: pre-existing renal impairment
  renal artery stenosis
  taking non-steroidal anti-inflammatory drugs
  taking a diuretic

- **Hyperkalaemia**

- **Cough**

  Headache, nausea, diarrhoea, pancreatitis, blood dyscrasias, skin rashes, itching, peripheral neuropathy and photosensitivity, as well as angioneurotic oedema, have all been reported, but are uncommon.

Table 14
Side-effects of ACE inhibitors.

ACE inhibitors can cause impairment of renal function which may progress and become severe. At particular risk are those with pre-existing renal impairment, and ACE inhibitors should be used with caution in those with a serum creatinine >150 mmol/l and, if possible, not at all in those with a serum creatinine >200 mmol/l.

Renal failure may also be aggravated by the concomitant prescription of non-steroidal anti-inflammatory drugs or diuretics. Patients with peripheral vascular disease or generalized atherosclerosis may have silent atherosclerotic renal artery stenosis. ACE inhibitors should be used with particular caution in these patients as renal failure may be precipitated. Serum urea and electrolytes should be checked in all patients prior to initiating therapy with ACE inhibitors and at regular intervals thereafter.

α-adrenoceptor blockers

The antihypertensive effect of α-blockers is mediated by peripheral vasodilation and hence a reduction in peripheral vascular resistance. However, non-selective agents also cause a reflex tachycardia. Selective α_1-blockers such as prazosin avoid the reflex tachycardia but still appear to cause significant postural hypotension – probably due to their effects on venous dilatation. This has limited their use in the elderly as they are particularly prone to postural hypotension.

Newer α_1-blocking drugs such as doxazosin and terazosin have fewer reported effects on postural hypotension. They have no adverse effects on renal function and have recently been shown to be useful in the management of benign prostatic hypertrophy, improving prostatic symptoms. They are also a useful adjunct to the treatment of cardiac failure.

Other antihypertensives

The older antihypertensive treatments such as methyldopa and clonidine, which have a central anti-adrenergic effect, have now been largely superseded. Methyldopa can cause postural hypotension, Coombes-positive haemolytic anaemia, liver dysfunction, confusion and depression. Clonidine can aggravate cardiac failure and cause depression, as well as causing possibly dangerous rebound hypertension if doses are omitted, i.e. patients forget to take their tablets.

Compliance

In any age group, a common cause of treatment failure is poor compliance. Most hypertensive patients are asymptomatic and may fail to appreciate the potential benefits of treatment, particularly if drug regimens are complicated or cause side-effects.

The simpler the treatment the more likely the patient is to comply with therapy (Table 15). The best compliance occurs with a regimen of one tablet a day, or at most a B.D. dose.

- Clear explanation of dose and timing
- Information regarding possible adverse effects, their significance and duration
- Patients know why they are taking the tablets and what the benefits are
- Avoiding complicated treatment schedule – once daily or B.D. doses preferred
- Avoiding long waiting times in the doctor's surgery and poor transportation facilities between the patient's home and the surgery or hospital
- Involving family/carers, particularly if poor memory is a problem

Table 15
Factors improving compliance.

Drug interactions

Elderly patients are often taking other prescribed medications or 'over the counter' preparations. These may interact with antihypertensive agents leading to either increased toxicity, or potentiation or antagonism of the antihypertensive effect. An example of this is the potential interaction between nifedipine and cimetidine which is now available 'over the counter'. This may lead to raised plasma concentrations of nifedipine, possibly leading to an increased risk of side-effects. The following outlines some of the common drug interactions which must be borne in mind when prescribing for elderly patients:

Drugs that potentiate antihypertensive effects

- Antipsychotic agents, especially phenothiazine
- Antidepressants, especially tricyclics
- L-dopa preparations
- Benzodiapezines
- Baclofen
- Alcohol

Drugs that antagonise antihypertensive effects

- Corticosteroids
- Non-steroidal anti-inflammatory drugs

Specific interactions leading to toxicity

Thiazide diuretics

• Theophyllines, steroids or β-agonists	↑ risk of hypokalaemia ↓ excretion
• Lithium	↑ risk of toxicity
• Carbamazepine	↑ risk of hyponatraemia

β-blockers

• Verapamil	possible bradycardia, asystole, hypotension, heart failure
• Digoxin	profound bradycardia
• Oral hypoglycaemics	enhanced hypoglycaemic effects, mask the warning signs of hypoglycaemia

Calcium antagonists

- Tricyclic antidepressants
  (imipramine)

  ↑ plasma concentrations
  when given with
  diltiazem or verapamil

- Lithium

  possible neurotoxicity
  with diltiazem or
  verapamil

- Digoxin

  levels ↑ by verapamil,
  diltiazem, nicardipine
  and nifedipine

- Phenytoin

  levels ↑ with diltiazem
  and nifedipine

ACE inhibitors

- Non-steroidal anti-inflammatory drugs   risk of renal failure

- Potassium-sparing diuretics   hyperkalaemia

- Cyclosporin   hyperkalaemia

- Digoxin   ↑ plasma concentrations

- Lithium   ↑ plasma concentrations

Quality of life and prevention of target organ damage

Most trials of antihypertensive drugs have resulted in withdrawal rates of 16–33% due to adverse effects. Many more patients, however, may experience mild side-effects which are not reported and do not lead to drug withdrawal. In particular patients may under-report subtle psychological changes such as effects on mood, memory and concentration, or sexual dysfunction. Although thiazides and β-blockers are well recognized to cause male sexual dysfunction, and lipophilic β-blockers in particular have been implicated in affecting memory and depression, at present there is a paucity of quality of life data specific to elderly patients on antihypertensive treatment. More work needs to be done in this area, particularly with the newer antihypertensives, if a particular drug is to be recommended in terms of a better effect on psychological functioning and quality of life.

Conclusion

Ideally, antihypertensive therapy should not only lower blood pressure but should prevent or improve end-organ damage. Some newer antihypertensive agents (e.g. calcium antagonists, ACE inhibitors) reduce left ventricular hypertrophy and maintain or improve renal blood flow. However, little is known of the effects of these newer agents on long-term morbidity and mortality. Further research will indicate in future whether these agents are of particular value in the prevention of morbidity and mortality from target-organ disease.

Conclusions

There is no doubt that hypertension is a major public health problem in the elderly, as at all ages. Evidence continues to accumulate concerning the benefits of treatment in the 'younger' old; and even in the very elderly the evidence is suggestive of benefit, although trials currently underway, such as the Hypertension in the Very Elderly Trial (HYVET), will shed more light on this matter.

In those under 80 years of age, it is the authors' practice to treat hypertension, be it systolic (systolic blood pressure >160 mmHg on three occasions) or diastolic/mixed (systolic blood pressure >160 mmHg and/or diastolic blood pressure >90 mmHg on three occasions) when there are no contraindications. Even in those over 80, we would consider offering treatment to those with hypertension, especially if they are 'biologically' young.

While non-pharmacological treatments and modifications of other risk factors would be offered first, the majority of treatments will inevitably involve antihypertensive drugs. A small dose of bendrofluazide (for example 2.5 mg daily) or similar thiazide would be our drug of first choice. If control is inadequate we would consider adding a small dose of a β-blocker such as atenolol (25 or 50 mg), although co-existing pathology in many elderly people may preclude the use of such drugs.

Calcium channel blockers such as inherently long-acting amlodipine (5–10 mg once daily) are unquestionably effective in reducing blood pressure and would be considered; recent concerns have been raised, however, regarding the effects of short-acting calcium channel blockers on overall cardiovascular safety. ACE inhibitors are effective and relatively safe, although they require careful monitoring in the early stages, may result in first dose hypotension, and must be used with extreme caution in those with renal impairment. These drugs are, however, particularly beneficial in those hypertensives with co-existing cardiac impairment.

Finally, it must be emphasized that the elderly population is very heterogeneous. Some chronologically old people are biologically very young; some younger people are biologically very old. The decision whether to treat and the choice of drugs must, as always in medicine, be made after careful consideration of the patient as an individual, not simply as someone who happens to have been born a very long time ago.

Further reading

Amery A, Brixko P, Clement D, et al. Mortality and morbidity results from the European Working Party in High Blood Pressure in the Elderly trial. *Lancet* 1985;**i**:1349–1354.

Amery A, Birkenhager W, Brixko P, et al. Efficacy of antihypertensive drug treatment according to age, sex, blood pressure and previous cardiovascular disease in patients over the age of 60. *Lancet* 1986;**ii**:589–592.

Applegate WB. Hypertension in elderly patients. *Annals of Internal Medicine* 1989;**110**:901–915.

Byyny RL. Hypertension in the elderly. In: Laragh JH, Brenner BM (Eds). *Hypertension: Pathophysiology, Diagnosis and Management.* Raven Press, New York 1990: pp 1869–1887.

Chobanian AV. Pathophysiologic considerations in the treatment of the elderly hypertensive patient. *American Journal of Cardiology* 1983;**52**:49D–53D.

Coope J, Warrender TS. Randomised trial of treatment of hypertension in elderly patients in primary care. *British Medical Journal* 1986;**293**:1145–1151.

Cornoni-Huntley JC, LaCroix AZ, Havlik RJ. Race and sex differentials in the impact of hypertension in the United States: the National Health and Nutrition Examination Survey. I. Epidemiologic follow-up survey. *Archives of Internal Medicine* 1989;**149**:780–788.

Dahlof B, Lindholm LH, Hansson L, et al. Morbidity and morality in the Swedish Trial of Old Patients with Hypertension (STOP–Hypertension). *Lancet* 1991;**338**:1281–1285.

Emeriau JP. What is the clinical relevance of isolated systolic hypertension? *Drugs and Aging* 1992;**2**:147–152.

Farnett L, Mulrow CD, Linn WD, Lucey CR, Tuley MR. The J-curve phenomenon and the treatment of hypertension. *Journal of the American Medical Association* 1991;**265**:489–495.

Harris T, Cook EF, Kannel WB, Goldman L. Proportional hazards analysis of risk factors for coronary heart disease in individuals aged 65 or older. *Journal of the American Geriatrics Society* 1988;**36**;1023–1028.

Hollenberg NK, Adams DF, Solomon RS, et al. Senecence and the renal vasculature in normal man. *Circulation Research* 1974;**34**:309–316.

Hypertension Detection and Follow-up Program Cooperative Group. Five year findings of the hypertension detection and follow-up program: I. Reduction in mortality of persons with high blood pressure, including mild hypertension; II. Mortality by race, sex and age. *Journal of the American Medical Association* 1979;**242**:2562–2571.

Jenkins AC, Knill JR, Dreslinski GR. Captopril in the treatment of the elderly hypertensive patient. *Archives of Internal Medicine* 1985;**145**:2029–2031.

Joint National Committee. Hypertension prevalence and the status of awareness treatment and Control in the United States: final report of the Sub-committee on Definition and Prevalence of the 1984 Joint National Committee. *Hypertension* 1985;**7**:457–468.

Kannel WB, Gordon T. Evaluation of cardiovascular risk in the elderly: the Framingham study. *Bulletin of the New York Academy of Medicine* 1978;**54**:573–591.

Kannel WB, Dawber TR, McGee DL. Perspectives on systolic hypertension: the Framingham study. *Circulation* 1980;**6**:1179–1182.

Kaplan NM. Non-drug treatment of hypertension. *Annals of Internal Medicine* 1985;**102**:359–373.

Lakatta EG. Mechanisms of hypertension in the elderly. *Journal of the American Geriatrics Society* 1989;**37**:780–790.

Langer RD, Ganiats TG, Barrett-Conner E. Paradoxical survival of elderly men with high blood pressure. *British Medical Journal* 1989;**298**:1356–1358.

Lindeman RD, Tobin J, Shock NW. Longitudinal studies in rate of decline in renal function with age. *Journal of the American Geriatrics Society* 1985;**33**:278–285.

Lowenstein FW. Blood pressure in relation to age and sex in the tropics and subtropics: a review of the literature and an investigation in two tribes of Brazil Indians. *Lancet* 1961;**i**:389–392.

Master AM, Lasser RP, Jaffe HL. Blood pressure in white people over 65 years of age. *Annals of Internal Medicine* 1958;**48**:284–290.

Mattila K, Haavisto M, Rajala S, Heikenheimo R. Blood pressure and five year survival in the very old. *British Medical Journal* 1988;**296**:887–889.

Messerli FH, Sundgaard-Riise K, Ventura HO, et al. Essential hypertension in the elderly: hemodynamics, intravascular volume, plasma renin activity, and circulating catecholamine levels. *Lancet* 1983;**ii**:983–986.

MRC Working Party. Medical Research Council trial of treatment of hypertension in older adults. *British Medical Journal* 1992;**304**:405–412.

Mulkerrin EC, Brain A, Hampton D, et al. Reduced renal hemodynamic response to atrial natriuretic peptide in elderly volunteers. *American Journal of Kidney Diseases* 1993;**22**:538–544.

Multiple Risk Factor Intervention Trial Research Group. Multiple risk factor intervention trial – risk factor changes and mortality results. *Journal of the American Medical Association* 1982;**248**:1465–1476.

Noth RH, Lassman MN, Tan SY, Fernandez-Cruz Jr A, Mulrow PJ. Age and the renin–aldosterone system. *Archives of Internal Medicine* 1977;**137**:1414–1417.

Robertson JIS. Hypertension and its treatment in the elderly. *Clinical and Experimental Hypertension* 1989;**11**:779–805.

Rowe JW, Troen BR. Sympathetic nervous system and aging man. *Endocrine Reviews* 1980;**1**:167–178.

Savage DS, Garrison RJ, Kannel WB, et al. The spectrum of left ventricular hypertrophy in a general population sample: the Framingham study. *Circulation* 1987;**75 (Suppl.1)**:26–33.

Scott P, Giese J. Age and the renin–angiotensin system. *Acta Medica Scandinavia* 1983;**676 (Suppl)**:45–51.

SHEP Cooperative Research Group. Rationale and design of a randomized clinical trial on prevention of stroke in isolated systolic hypertension. *Journal of Clinical Epidemiology* 1988;**41**:1197–1208.

SHEP Cooperative Research Group. Prevention of stroke by antihypertensive drug treatment in older persons with isolated systolic hypertension. *Journal of the American Medical Association* 1991;**265**:3255–3264.

Topol EJ, Traill TA, Fortuin NG. Hypertensive hypertrophic cardiomyopathy of the elderly. *New England Journal of Medicine* 1985;**312**:277–283.

Vestal RE, Wood AJ, Shand DG. Reduced β-adrenoceptor sensitivity in the elderly. *Clinical Pharmacology and Therapeutics* 1979;**26**:181–186.

Whelton PK, Klag ML. Epidemiology of high blood pressure. *Clinics in Geriatric Medicine* 1989;**5**:639–655.

Working Group on Hypertension in the Elderly. Statement on hypertension in the elderly. *Journal of the American Medical Association* 1986;**256**:70–74.

Index

Page numbers in *italic* refer to the illustrations